Geneva Fern

Ageless Strength: Mastering Life with Daily Exercise Rituals for Lifelong Vitality

This book was professionally typeset on Reedsy
Find out more at reedsy.com

To all those who embrace the boundless journey of age, defying limitations and embracing the strength within. May these pages inspire you to transcend perceived boundaries, nurture the flame of vitality, and revel in the joy of lifelong wellness. Here's to rewriting the narrative of ageing, one resilient step at a time.

Contents

    1.

    2.

    3.

    4.

    5.

    6.

    7.

    8.

    9.

10.

11.

12.

Foreword

Imagine opening the book "Ageless Strength" and stepping into a world where age is not a limitation but a gateway to lasting vitality.

Preface

In a world that often celebrates the exuberance of youth, the true essence of strength and vitality can transcend the barriers of age. Welcome to "Ageless Strength," a journey that defies the conventional notions of ageing, inviting you to discover the boundless potential of your body, regardless of the years that have passed.

This book is a testament to the human spirit's indomitable capacity for growth and transformation. It beckons you to shatter the limitations you've placed upon yourself and embrace a life brimming with vigour and energy. Whether you're in your twenties or beyond your sixties, the principles outlined within these pages hold the power to rejuvenate your body, mind, and spirit.

As the years accumulate, it's tempting to resign to the notion that our best physical days are behind us. The aches and pains become part of our daily narrative, and the mirror reflects a version of ourselves we're less acquainted with. But let me assure you, this need not be your narrative.

"Ageless Strength" is not just a fitness guide; it's a philosophy that challenges the very fabric of how we perceive ageing. Within these chapters, you'll find a treasure trove of knowledge and guidance. You'll uncover the secrets of exercises that fortify your body's foundation, foster resilience, and invite the joy of movement back into your life. From the simple elegance of foundational exercises to the intricacies of integrating strength with cardiovascular endurance, every chapter offers a stepping stone toward your fountain of vitality.

But "Ageless Strength" is more than sets and reps. It's a holistic approach that extends its reach to embrace the interconnectedness of your being. Mobility, flexibility, and core stability weave seamlessly into your journey, enhancing not just your physical prowess, but also your quality of life. This book recognizes the importance of recovery, offering you the wisdom to heal and prevent injuries, ensuring that every stride of progress is made on solid ground.

Ageing isn't a journey to be feared or merely endured; it's an expedition to be embraced and celebrated. "Ageless Strength" empowers you to reclaim your strength, your confidence, and your vitality. It's a reminder that the story of your body is far from over, and every chapter yet to be written holds the promise of newfound vigour.

So, turn the page and embark on this transformative voyage. Let the words on these pages be the catalyst for a revolution in the way you perceive your body and its capabilities. With "Ageless Strength" as your guide, you'll find that the journey toward vitality is timeless, and the destination is within your grasp, regardless of the miles you've travelled.

1

Explanation of the importance of strength training for all ages.

Strength training is a form of exercise that involves using resistance to build and develop muscular strength, endurance, and size. It's commonly associated with weightlifting, but it can involve various types of resistance, including body weight, resistance bands, and free weights. The importance of strength training applies to individuals of all ages, from children to seniors, and here's **why:**

1. **Muscle Mass Preservation and Development**: As we age, there is a natural tendency for muscle mass to decrease, a condition known as sarcopenia. Strength training helps counteract this process by stimulating muscle growth and preservation. This is crucial for maintaining overall physical function and independence, as muscles play a key role in activities of daily living.

2. **Bone Health:** Strength training places stress on the bones, which prompts them to become stronger and denser. This is particularly important for preventing osteoporosis, a condition characterized by

fragile and brittle bones. Building strong bones during younger years can reduce the risk of fractures and other bone-related issues later in life.

3. **Metabolism Boost:** Muscles are metabolically active tissues, meaning they burn more calories even at rest compared to other types of tissue. By increasing muscle mass through strength training, you can boost your resting metabolic rate, making it easier to manage weight and overall body composition.

4. **Joint Health and Injury Prevention:** Strength training helps improve joint stability and range of motion. It also reinforces the ligaments and tendons surrounding the joints, reducing the risk of injuries and enhancing overall joint health.

5. **Functional Fitness**: Daily activities require strength and muscle endurance. Strength training improves your ability to perform tasks such as lifting, carrying, walking, and climbing stairs, making your daily life more manageable and enjoyable.

6. **Balance and Coordination:** Strong muscles are crucial for maintaining balance and coordination. This is especially significant as we age, as falls are a leading cause of injuries among older adults. Strength training helps enhance muscle control and balance, reducing the risk of falls.

7. **Hormonal Benefits**: Strength training triggers the release of hormones such as testosterone and growth hormone, which are

essential for muscle growth and overall vitality. These hormones play a role in various bodily functions beyond just muscle development.

8. **Mental Health**: Exercise, including strength training, has been linked to improved mental well-being. Physical activity releases endorphins, which are natural mood enhancers. Engaging in regular strength training can help reduce stress, anxiety, and depression.

9. **Quality of Life:** Maintaining strength and physical function directly impacts your quality of life. Being physically capable and independent enables you to engage in activities you love and maintain a higher level of autonomy as you age.

10. **Longevity**: Studies suggest that individuals who engage in regular strength training may experience improved longevity and a reduced risk of chronic diseases.

It's important to note that when starting any exercise program, including strength training, individuals of all ages should consult with a healthcare professional, especially if they have pre-existing health conditions. Strength training programs should be tailored to individual fitness levels and goals to ensure safety and effectiveness.

2

Getting Started: Assessing Your Fitness Level

Assessing your fitness level is a crucial step in any journey towards improved health and strength. This aims to guide you through a series of self-assessment tests that will help you understand your current physical capabilities. By gauging where you are at the beginning of your fitness regimen, you'll be better equipped to set realistic goals and track your progress over time.

<u>Understanding Your Baseline:</u>

Before embarking on any exercise program, it's important to establish a baseline. This involves evaluating your cardiovascular endurance, muscular strength, flexibility, and overall mobility. These components collectively contribute to your fitness level, and an accurate assessment will provide a clear starting point for your fitness journey.

<u>**Self-Assessment Tests:**</u>

This section delves into specific self-assessment tests that cover different aspects of fitness:

1. Cardiovascular Endurance Test

This test measures your body's ability to sustain aerobic exercise. A common method is the 1-mile walk test, where you briskly walk one mile while timing yourself. Your performance can indicate your cardiovascular health and potential areas for improvement.

2. Muscular Strength Test

Assess your muscle strength using exercises like push-ups, sit-ups, or squats. Count the number of repetitions you can perform with proper form. This helps you understand your muscular endurance and where you might need to focus on building strength.

3. Flexibility Test

Flexibility is crucial for preventing injuries and maintaining functional movement. The sit-and-reach test, where you measure how far you can stretch while seated, is a simple way to assess your flexibility.

4. Mobility Assessment

Mobility refers to your joints' range of motion. This can be evaluated through exercises like shoulder circles, hip rotations, and ankle movements. Identifying areas of restricted mobility will guide your flexibility and mobility training.

<u>**Recording Your Results:**</u>

After completing each self-assessment test, record your results in a fitness journal or a digital tracking tool. This serves as a snapshot of your initial fitness level. Documenting your starting point will help you track your progress as you move forward.

<u>**Interpreting Your Results;**</u>

Once you've completed the self-assessment tests and recorded your results, it's time to interpret what they mean:

- <u>**Identifying Strengths**</u>: Recognize areas where you excel. This could be above-average cardiovascular endurance, strong core muscles, or good flexibility.

- <u>**Pinpointing Weaknesses:**</u> Highlight areas that need improvement. Maybe your muscular strength is lower than desired or your flexibility is limited.

-**Setting Realistic Goals**: Based on your strengths and weaknesses, set achievable fitness goals. For instance, if your cardiovascular endurance is excellent but your flexibility is lacking, you might aim to incorporate more stretching routines into your regimen.

<u>**Consulting a Professional**</u>

While self-assessment tests provide valuable insights, consulting a fitness professional or healthcare provider is recommended, especially if you're new to exercise or have underlying health concerns. They can provide a more comprehensive evaluation and tailor recommendations to your individual needs.

3

The Basics: Foundation Exercises

Squats:

Squats are a fundamental compound exercise that targets the muscles of the lower body, primarily the quadriceps, hamstrings, and glutes. They also engage the core for stability. Here's a detailed explanation of how to perform squats correctly:

1. **Starting Position**: Stand with your feet shoulder-width apart. Keep your chest up, shoulders back, and core engaged. You can extend your arms forward for balance.

2. **Squatting Down**: Initiate the movement by pushing your hips back and bending your knees. Imagine sitting back in an imaginary chair. Ensure your knees don't go past your toes.

3. **Depth**: Lower yourself until your thighs are parallel to the ground or as low as your mobility allows. Keep your back straight and chest lifted throughout the movement.

4. **Pushing Up:** Push through your heels to return to the starting position, fully extending your hips and knees.

Lunges:

Lunges are excellent for developing lower body strength and balance. They primarily work the quads, hamstrings, and glutes. Here's how to perform a basic lunge:

1. **Starting Position**: Stand tall with your feet together and arms by your sides.

2. **Lunging**: Take a step forward with one leg and lower your body until both knees are bent at 90-degree angles. The back knee should hover slightly above the ground.

3. **Pushing Back:** Push off the front foot and step back to the starting position.

4. **Alternate Sides:** Repeat the movement with the opposite leg.

Push-Ups:

Push-ups are a classic bodyweight exercise that strengthens the chest, shoulders, triceps, and core. Here's how to perform a proper push-up:

1. **Starting Position**: Start in a high plank position with your hands slightly wider than shoulder-width apart. Your body should form a straight line from head to heels.

2. **Lowering:** Lower your body by bending your elbows. Keep your core engaged and your body in a straight line. Aim to lower until your chest is just above the ground.

3. **Pushing Up**: Push through your palms to extend your arms and return to the starting position.

Planks:

Planks are excellent for building core strength and stability. They engage the entire core and help improve posture. Here's how to perform a basic plank:

1. **Starting Position:** Begin in a high plank position, similar to the push-up position, with your hands directly under your shoulders.

2. **Alignment**: Keep your body in a straight line from head to heels. Engage your core, glutes, and leg muscles.

3. **Hold and Breathe**: Maintain this position, focusing on your breathing. Start with shorter durations (e.g., 20 seconds) and gradually increase as you get stronger.

4. **Variations:** To challenge yourself, try side planks (weight on one arm, body sideways), or forearm planks (resting on your forearms instead of hands).

Daily Exercise Routine:

- **Squats:** Perform 3 sets of 10-12 repetitions. Rest 1-2 minutes between sets.

- **Lunges:** Do 3 sets of 10 reps per leg. Rest 1-2 minutes between sets.

- **Push-Ups**: Aim for 3 sets of 8-10 repetitions. If regular push-ups are challenging, start with knee push-ups.

- **Planks:** Hold a plank for 20-30 seconds. Repeat 3 times with 30-60 seconds of rest between sets.

4

Full-Body Workouts: Daily Routine

Daily **Full-Body Workout Plan: Incorporating Various Muscle Groups:**

Warm-Up: 5-10 minutes

- Begin with 5-10 minutes of light cardio, such as brisk walking, jogging in place, or jumping jacks, to increase heart rate and warm up the muscles.

- Follow cardio with dynamic stretches, focusing on areas you'll be targeting during the workout. Examples include arm circles, leg swings, and hip rotations.

Main Workout:

1. **Squats** (Targets: Legs, Glutes, Core)

- Stand with feet shoulder-width apart.

- Lower your hips as if sitting in a chair, keeping your back straight and chest up.

- Push through your heels to return to the starting position.

- Aim for 3 sets of 12-15 reps.

2. **Push-Ups** (Targets: Chest, Shoulders, Triceps, Core)

   - Start in a plank position with hands slightly wider than shoulder-width apart.

   - Lower your body while keeping your core engaged and elbows close to your body.

   - Push back up to the starting position.

   - Perform 3 sets of 10-12 reps.

3. **Rows** (Targets: Back, Biceps, Shoulders)

   - Find a sturdy horizontal surface (like a table) at waist height.

   - Hold onto the edge of the surface and position yourself at an angle.

   - Pull your body toward the surface, leading with your elbows.

   - Lower yourself back down with control.

   - Complete 3 sets of 10-12 reps.

4. **Planks** (Targets: Core, Shoulders, Back)

   - Start in a push-up position, but rest on your forearms instead of your hands.

   - Keep your body in a straight line from head to heels, engaging your core.

   - Hold the position for as long as you can maintain proper form, aiming for 20-30 seconds initially.

5. **Lunges** (Targets: Legs, Glutes, Core)

   - Step forward with one leg and lower your body until both knees are at 90-degree angles.

- Push through the heel of your front foot to return to the starting position.

- Alternate legs and complete 3 sets of 10-12 reps per leg.

6. **Dips** (Targets: Triceps, Shoulders, Chest)

- Find parallel bars or use the edge of a stable surface.

- Lower your body by bending your elbows until your upper arms are parallel to the ground.

- Push back up to the starting position.

- Perform 3 sets of 10-12 reps.

Cool-Down: 5-10 minutes

- Finish with static stretches for major muscle groups, holding each stretch for 15-30 seconds.

- Incorporate deep breathing to aid in relaxation and recovery.

Progression and Adaptation:

Increase the resistance (weight or intensity) gradually as you become stronger.

Modify exercises if needed. For instance, beginners might do knee push-ups or assisted squats.

Aim to increase reps, sets, or time gradually to avoid plateaus.

Frequency and Rest:

Perform this full-body workout routine 3-4 times per week, with rest days in between to allow for muscle recovery.

<u>**Hydration and Nutrition:**</u>

Stay hydrated before, during, and after the workout. Consume a balanced meal or snack that includes carbohydrates and protein within an hour after the workout to aid recovery.

5

Cardio and Strength Integration

Cardiovascular Exercise: Cardio workouts, often referred to as aerobic exercises, elevate your heart rate and improve the efficiency of your cardiovascular system. These exercises include activities like running, cycling, swimming, and brisk walking. They help increase lung capacity, enhance circulation, and burn calories, ultimately improving your endurance and stamina.

Strategies for Cardiovascular and Strength Training Integration:

1. **Alternating Between Exercises:**
   - Alternate between cardiovascular exercises and strength exercises in a circuit-style workout. This keeps your heart rate elevated while giving your muscles a chance to recover between strength sets.

2. **High-Intensity Interval Training (HIIT):**
   - Incorporate HIIT workouts, which involve short bursts of intense cardiovascular exercises followed by brief rest periods. HIIT

effectively burns calories, boosts metabolism, and improves cardiovascular fitness.

3. **Compound Movements**:

- Choose strength exercises that engage multiple muscle groups simultaneously. These compound movements, like squats and deadlifts, elevate your heart rate while building strength.

4. **Supersets**:

- Pair strength exercises that target different muscle groups and perform them back-to-back with minimal rest. This approach keeps your heart rate up and optimizes workout efficiency.

5. **Cardio Between Sets:**

- Instead of resting completely between strength sets, perform a short burst of cardiovascular activity, such as jumping jacks or high knees, to maintain an elevated heart rate.

6. **Longer Workouts:**

- On certain days, opt for longer workouts that incorporate both steady-state cardiovascular exercise (e.g., jogging) and a comprehensive strength routine.

Daily Exercise Plan: Cardio and Strength Integration

Warm-up: 5-10 minutes of light cardiovascular activity (e.g., brisk walking, light jogging).

Circuit Workout (Repeat 3 Times)

1. **Jump Rope**: 2 minutes
2. **Squats**: 15 repetitions
3. **Push-Ups**: 12 repetitions
4. **Lunges**: 12 repetitions per leg
5. **Burpees:** 10 repetitions
6. **Dumbbell Rows**: 12 repetitions per arm
7. **Mountain Climbers**: 1 minute
8. **Plank**: Hold for 45 seconds

Cardiovascular Segment

- **Jogging**: 10 minutes at a moderate pace.
- **Sprinting:** 6 sets of 30-second sprints with 1-minute rest between each.

Strength Training Segment

1. **Bench Press:** 3 sets of 8 repetitions
2. **Deadlifts:** 3 sets of 8 repetitions
3. **Pull-Ups**: 3 sets of 6 repetitions
4. **Leg Press**: 3 sets of 10 repetitions

5. **Bicep Curls:** 3 sets of 12 repetitions

6. **Tricep Dips**: 3 sets of 12 repetitions

Cool-down: 5-10 minutes of static stretching for major muscle groups.

Important Notes:

- Always start with a proper warm-up to prevent injury.

- Hydration is crucial. Drink water throughout the workout.

- Focus on proper form to avoid injury and achieve optimal results.

- Adjust the intensity and repetitions according to your fitness level.

- Consider incorporating a variety of cardio activities, such as cycling or swimming, to keep things interesting.

6

Mobility and Flexibility

Mobility and flexibility are essential components of physical fitness that often receive less attention than strength and cardiovascular conditioning. However, they play a crucial role in maintaining a well-rounded and functional body. Mobility refers to the ability to move a joint actively through its full range of motion, while flexibility is the passive lengthening of a muscle. These aspects contribute to overall movement quality, joint health, and injury prevention.

Daily Exercise Routine for Mobility and Flexibility:

Incorporating daily exercises for mobility and flexibility can have a transformative impact on your overall well-being. This routine is designed to be simple yet effective, helping you gradually improve your range of motion and muscle flexibility over time. Remember to perform each exercise in a controlled manner and never push yourself to the point of pain.

Exercise 1: Neck Rotations (2 minutes)

Gently rotate your neck in a circular motion, starting with slow, small rotations and gradually increasing the range. Perform 10 rotations in each direction.

Exercise 2: Shoulder Circles (3 minutes)

Stand with your arms relaxed at your sides. Slowly raise your shoulders, roll them back, and lower them down in a circular motion. Perform 10 circles forward and then 10 circles backwards.

Exercise 3: Cat-Cow Stretch (4 minutes)

Assume a tabletop position on your hands and knees. Inhale as you arch your back, lifting your tailbone and head (cow pose). Exhale as you round your spine, tucking your chin to your chest (cat pose). Repeat this sequence for 2 minutes.

Exercise 4: Hip Flexor Stretch (3 minutes per side)

Step into a lunge position, with one leg forward and the other extended behind you. Gently press your hips forward while keeping your back straight to stretch the hip flexors. Hold for 30 seconds on each side.

Exercise 5: Standing Forward Fold (3 minutes)

Stand with your feet hip-width apart. Slowly bend at your hips, letting your upper body hang toward the ground. Let your head and neck relax. Hold this stretch for 3 minutes, allowing your muscles to gradually release tension.

Exercise 6: Hamstring Stretch (2 minutes per side)

Sit on the floor with one leg extended straight and the other bent, sole against your inner thigh. Reach toward your extended foot, keeping your back straight. Hold for 1 minute on each side.

Exercise 7: Quadriceps Stretch (2 minutes per side)

Stand near a wall or support for balance. Grab one ankle and gently pull it toward your glutes, feeling a stretch in the front of your thigh. Hold for 1 minute on each side.

Exercise 8: Spinal Twist (3 minutes per side)

Lie on your back and bring one knee toward your chest. Let it fall across your body, extending your opposite arm out to the side. Gently twist your spine while looking in the opposite direction. Hold for 1.5 minutes on each side.

Exercise 9: Ankle Circles (2 minutes per side)

Sit on the floor with your legs extended. Lift one foot off the ground and rotate your ankle in a circular motion. Perform 10 circles in each direction before switching to the other ankle.

Exercise 10: Deep Breathing and Meditation (5 minutes)

End your routine with deep, slow breaths. Inhale deeply through your nose, expand your lungs fully, and exhale slowly through your mouth. Spend a few minutes in meditation, focusing on your improved mobility and flexibility and cultivating a sense of relaxation.

Incorporating Mobility and Flexibility into Your Day:

1. **Morning Stretches:** Begin your day with a few gentle stretches.

Upon waking up, spend a few minutes performing simple stretches in bed. Focus on elongating your body, stretching your arms overhead, and gently rotating your ankles and wrists. These gentle movements help to awaken your muscles and increase blood flow.

2. **Desk or Office Stretches**: Counteract the effects of prolonged sitting.

If you have a desk job, make a conscious effort to take short breaks throughout the day. Every hour, stand up and perform stretches to counteract the effects of sitting. Neck stretches, seated twists, and shoulder rolls are excellent options. These quick stretches help prevent stiffness and promote blood circulation.

3. **Lunchtime Walks**: Combine movement and fresh air.

Use your lunch break as an opportunity to go for a walk. Walking not only improves cardiovascular health but also enhances joint mobility. Walk briskly and swing your arms to engage your upper body. If possible, find a park or green space to enjoy nature while moving your body.

4. **Post-Work Stretching**: Wind down after a day of activity.

When you return home, dedicate a few minutes to stretching. Focus on areas that tend to tense up during the day, such as your shoulders, hips, and lower back. This can help release tension accumulated from daily activities.

5. **Incorporate Yoga or Pilates**: Join a class or practice at home.

Consider joining a yoga or Pilates class or practising at home. These disciplines emphasize both mobility and flexibility through flowing movements and poses. They also incorporate breathing techniques that promote relaxation and reduce stress.

6. **Evening Mobility Routine**: Prepare your body for rest.

Before bed, engage in a gentle mobility routine. This can include movements like hip circles, spinal twists, and ankle rotations. This routine not only improves flexibility but also helps your body relax before sleep.

7. **Hydration and Nutrition**: Support joint health from within.

Staying hydrated is essential for maintaining joint health and overall flexibility. Drink plenty of water throughout the day. Additionally, include foods rich in antioxidants, Omega-3 fatty acids, and nutrients like vitamin D and calcium to support your joints and muscles.

8. **Mindful Breathing**: Enhance relaxation and flexibility.

Incorporate deep breathing and mindfulness techniques into your day. Deep breaths provide oxygen to your muscles and help you stay relaxed, which can enhance your flexibility. Consider setting aside a few minutes during breaks to close your eyes, take deep breaths, and clear your mind.

9. **Weekend Active Recovery**: Embrace active leisure time.

On weekends, engage in activities that promote mobility and flexibility. Go for longer walks, try hiking, or explore gentle forms of exercise like swimming or cycling. These activities contribute to your overall mobility while allowing you to enjoy your free time.

10. **Regular Self-Assessment:** Monitor your progress.

Periodically assess your mobility and flexibility improvements. Take note of how certain stretches have become easier and how your range of motion has increased. This self-awareness can be motivating and help you adjust your routine as needed.

7

Core Strength and Stability

T**he Core Muscles Explained:**

The core is composed of various muscles, including the rectus abdominis, obliques, transverse abdominis, erector spinae, and more. Each muscle plays a unique role in maintaining stability, facilitating movement, and providing support to the entire body. The rectus abdominis, for instance, aids in flexing the spine, while the transverse abdominis acts as a natural weight belt, enhancing spinal stability.

Benefits of a Strong Core:

1. **Posture Improvement**: A strong core helps maintain a proper alignment of the spine, reducing the risk of poor posture-related issues such as back pain and discomfort.
2. **Enhanced Balance**: Core muscles enable better balance and coordination by stabilizing the body during various movements, preventing falls and injuries.

3. **Functional Strength**: Many everyday tasks involve core engagement. Strengthening these muscles translates to improved performance in daily activities.

4. **Injury Prevention:** A stable core acts as a shield, safeguarding the spine and other vulnerable areas from strains and injuries.

5. **Athletic Performance**: Core strength is a cornerstone of athletic prowess, contributing to efficient energy transfer and controlled movements.

Daily Core Exercise Routine:

Warm-Up:

Before diving into the core exercises, it's important to warm up your body to increase blood flow and prepare your muscles for the workout. You can spend about 5-10 minutes on light cardio, such as brisk walking, light jogging, or jumping jacks. Follow this with dynamic stretches like hip circles, leg swings, and torso twists.

Plank Variations:

1. **Standard Plank (30 seconds):** Get into a push-up position with your hands directly under your shoulders and your body forming a straight line from head to heels. Engage your core, glutes, and quads while keeping your neck in line with your spine. Hold this position

for 30 seconds, focusing on maintaining a strong core and steady breathing.

2. **Side Planks (20 seconds on each side):** Lie on your side, legs stacked, and prop yourself up on your elbow. Keep your body in a straight line and engage your obliques. Hold this position for 20 seconds on each side. To make it more challenging, raise your top leg while in the side plank position.

3. **Plank with Leg Lifts (20 seconds for each leg)**: Start in a standard plank position. Lift one leg a few inches off the ground while maintaining a stable core and neutral spine. Alternate legs for 20 seconds each. This exercise challenges both your core stability and balance.

Crunches:

1. **Basic Crunches (20 reps)**: Lie on your back with your knees bent and feet flat on the floor. Place your hands lightly behind your head, elbows out to the sides. Engage your core and lift your upper body off the ground, aiming to bring your shoulder blades towards your knees. Lower back down with control.

2. **Reverse Crunches (20 reps)**: Lie on your back with your legs lifted off the ground, knees bent at 90 degrees. Lift your hips off the ground while curling your knees towards your chest. This targets the lower abdominal muscles.

Russian Twists (20 reps):

Sit on the ground with your knees bent and feet lifted off the ground. Hold a weight or your hands together. Lean back slightly while maintaining a straight back. Twist your torso to the right and then to the left, tapping the weight of your hands on the ground beside you for each twist.

Leg Raises (15 reps):

Lie on your back with your legs straight. Place your hands under your hips for support. Lift your legs off the ground while keeping them straight. Lower them back down slowly without letting them touch the floor.

Cool-Down:

After completing the core exercises, cool down with static stretches to release tension in the muscles you've worked. Perform stretches like Child's Pose, Cat-Cow, and Cobra Pose to gently stretch your core and back muscles.

Progression and Modifications in Core Strength Training:

Advancing your core strength and stability requires a systematic approach that gradually challenges your muscles while maintaining safety and proper form. This subchapter outlines effective methods of progression and offers modifications to ensure your core exercises remain engaging and effective over time.

<u>Progression Strategies:</u>

1. **Increased Time Under Tension:** One straightforward way to progress is by increasing the time you spend performing each exercise. For example, if you start with a 30-second plank, aim to extend it to 45 seconds or a minute as you become more comfortable.

2. **Add Resistance**: Incorporate light weights or resistance bands into traditional exercises like crunches or Russian twists. Holding a weight during exercises increases the load on your core muscles, promoting strength gains.

3. **Complex Movements**: Combine different core exercises into a sequence. For instance, perform a plank, followed by mountain climbers, and then a side plank. This challenges your core in various ways and encourages coordination.

4. **Unstable Surfaces**: Performing core exercises on unstable surfaces like a stability ball or Bosu ball engages additional stabilizing muscles, intensifying the workout.

5. **Elevated Legs**: Elevating your legs during exercises like leg raises or reverse crunches adds difficulty by increasing the leverage and demand on your core muscles.

Modifications for Different Fitness Levels:

1. **Beginners**:

- Start with shorter durations and fewer repetitions for each exercise.

- If full planks are challenging, perform modified planks on your knees or against a wall.

- For crunches, focus on the movement's quality rather than height.

2. **Intermediate**:

- Increase the intensity by incorporating standard planks, side planks, and other variations.

- Experiment with lifting one leg during planks or leg raises to engage the core differently.

- Gradually add weights or resistance bands to your exercises.

3. **Advanced**:

- Extend exercise durations, striving for 60-second planks and more challenging variations.

- Incorporate dynamic movements like bicycle crunches or hanging leg raises.

- Introduce advanced equipment like an ab wheel for rollouts.

Listening to Your Body:

Progression is essential, but not at the expense of safety or proper technique. Listen to your body and avoid pushing too hard, too quickly. Muscle soreness is expected, but sharp pain or discomfort should not be part of your routine. If an exercise causes pain, consider consulting a fitness professional or a healthcare provider.

Balancing Core Work with Rest:

Like any muscle group, your core muscles need time to recover. Integrate rest days into your routine to allow your core muscles to repair and strengthen. Overtraining can lead to injury and hinder progress.

Tracking Progress:

Keep a workout journal or use a fitness app to document your exercises, durations, and any modifications or advancements you make. Tracking your progress helps you stay accountable and motivated, and it allows you to celebrate your achievements.

8

Functional Strength for Daily Life

Enhancing Everyday Movement Patterns: The Essence of Functional Strength

1. **Real-World Relevance:** Functional strength training revolves around the idea that the exercises you do should mimic the movements you encounter regularly. This could involve actions like lifting, twisting, reaching, bending, and walking. By training your body to handle these movements more effectively, you're preparing yourself for the physical demands of your daily routines.

2. **Muscle Synergy**: Everyday tasks rarely isolate a single muscle group. For example, picking up a bag of groceries involves your legs, core, and arms working together. Functional exercises focus on multiple muscle groups simultaneously, encouraging them to coordinate and work in harmony. This synergy is crucial for efficient and injury-free movement.

3. **Balance and Stability:** Functional movements often require balance and stability. Think about maintaining your balance while

stepping off a curb or walking on an uneven surface. Functional exercises challenge your body's balance and stability mechanisms, ultimately improving your overall coordination and reducing the risk of falls.

4. **Improved Posture:** Functional strength training promotes good posture by targeting the muscles responsible for maintaining an upright stance. This can translate into better alignment during daily activities, leading to reduced strain on your spine and supporting structures.

5. **Core Strength:** A strong core is the foundation of many functional movements. Whether you're picking up a child or reaching for something high up, a stable core is essential. Functional exercises engage your core muscles, leading to improved core strength and stability.

6. **Injury Prevention**: By training your body to handle the movements you regularly perform, you're decreasing the risk of injury. When your muscles and joints are accustomed to these motions, they're less likely to be strained or injured when you perform them in real life.

7. **Maintaining Independence**: Functional strength training is especially valuable as you age. It helps maintain your ability to perform daily activities independently, which contributes to your overall quality of life and reduces the need for assistance.

- **Squatting:** Functional exercises like squats can improve your ability to get up from a chair, out of bed, or off the ground.

- **Lifting**: Incorporating deadlift variations can help you lift objects from the floor safely, reducing strain on your back.

- **Carrying**: Farmer's walks or carrying sandbags replicate carrying groceries, luggage, or other heavy objects.

- **Reaching**: Lunge and reach exercises enhance your flexibility and ability to reach high or low objects.

- **Twisting**: Core rotation exercises prepare your body for movements like looking over your shoulder while driving.

Functional Fitness: Beyond the Gym

Functional fitness is a training approach that goes beyond traditional gym workouts to prepare your body for the practical demands of daily life. It's about improving your ability to perform everyday movements efficiently and safely. Unlike exercises that isolate individual muscles, functional fitness focuses on training multiple muscle groups to work together harmoniously. This approach not only builds strength but also enhances coordination, balance, and mobility. The ultimate goal of functional fitness is to make your body more capable and resilient in real-world scenarios.

The Importance of Functional Fitness:

While traditional weightlifting and cardiovascular exercises are valuable for overall health, they might not fully prepare you for the specific movements you encounter in your daily routine. Functional fitness bridges this gap by targeting the movements you use regularly, such as bending, lifting, twisting, reaching, and walking. These movements might seem simple, but they often form the basis of our daily activities.

As we age, maintaining functional fitness becomes increasingly important. It can significantly impact our quality of life by preventing injuries, improving posture, and enabling us to stay independent. Whether you're picking up a child, carrying groceries, or getting in and out of a car, functional fitness helps ensure you can do so with ease and confidence.

Exercise Example: Functional Squat

Functional Movement Targeted: Rising from a chair or getting out of a car.

The functional squat exercise helps you build strength in your legs, glutes, and core muscles. It closely mimics the motion of getting up from a chair or standing up from a low position.

How to Perform a Functional Squat:

1. **Starting Position:** Stand with your feet shoulder-width apart, toes pointing slightly outward. Keep your chest up and your spine in a neutral position.

2. **Initiate the Squat:** Imagine you're about to sit in a chair. Lower your hips down and back as if you're sitting back in an imaginary chair. Your knees should bend and track over your toes.

3. **Keep Your Back Straight**: Maintain a straight back throughout the movement. Avoid rounding or arching your spine.

4. **Depth**: Aim to lower yourself until your thighs are approximately parallel to the ground. If you're comfortable, you can go deeper but don't force it.

5. **Rise:** Press through your heels to stand back up, extending your hips and knees.

6. **Repeat**: Perform several repetitions, focusing on a controlled motion and proper form.

Daily Functional Strength Routine:

This routine is designed to improve your functional fitness by targeting muscle groups and movement patterns commonly used in everyday activities. By incorporating these exercises into your daily routine, you'll develop the strength, mobility, and coordination necessary to perform daily tasks more easily and with reduced risk of injury. Remember to perform each exercise with proper form and control. If you're new to exercise, consider seeking guidance from a fitness professional before starting this routine.

1. **Squat to Chair Lifts:**

   - **Purpose**: This exercise mimics the action of getting up from a chair, which is a fundamental movement in daily life.

   - **How to Perform:**

   - Stand in front of a sturdy chair with your feet shoulder-width apart.

   - Lower your hips back and down into a squatting position, as if you were sitting down in the chair.

   - Press through your heels to stand back up without using your hands for assistance.

   - **Muscles Targeted**: Quadriceps, hamstrings, glutes.

2. **Farmer's Walk:**

   - **Purpose:** This exercise improves grip strength, overall body stability, and the ability to carry heavy objects.

   - **How to Perform**:

   - Hold a dumbbell or heavy object in each hand at your sides.

- Maintain an upright posture and engage your core.

- Take short and controlled steps while walking forward.

- **Muscles Targeted**: Forearms, grip strength, core, legs.

3. **Lunge and Reach:**

- **Purpose:** Replicating movements like reaching for items on high shelves or picking up objects from the ground.

- **How to Perform**:

- Start by standing with your feet together.

- Take a step forward into a lunge position, bending both knees.

- As you lower into the lunge, simultaneously reach one arm diagonally across your body.

- Return to the starting position and repeat on the other side.

- **Muscles Targeted**: Quadriceps, hamstrings, glutes, core, shoulders.

4. **Core Rotation with Resistance Band:**

- **Purpose**: Enhancing your ability to twist your torso, important for tasks like looking over your shoulder.

- **How to Perform**:

- Attach a resistance band at chest height.

- Hold the band's handle with both hands and stand perpendicular to the anchor point.

- Keep your hips stable and rotate your torso away from the anchor point while holding the band.

- Slowly return to the starting position and repeat on the other side.

- **Muscles Targeted:** Obliques, core, back.

5. **Step-Ups:**

- **<u>Purpose:</u>** This exercise improves leg strength, balance, and coordination, which are essential for activities like climbing stairs.

- **<u>How to Perform:</u>**

- Find a stable platform or step.

- Place one foot on the platform and push through the heel to step up.

- Bring the opposite knee up toward your chest.

- Step back down and repeat on the other side.

- **<u>Muscles Targeted:</u>** Quadriceps, hamstrings, glutes, calves.

<u>Incorporating the Routine:</u>

Perform this routine 2-3 times per week, allowing at least a day of rest between sessions. Start with 2 sets of 10-12 repetitions for each exercise and gradually increase the sets, reps, or resistance as you become more comfortable. Always prioritize proper form over the amount of weight or reps. Over time, you'll notice improvements in your strength, stability, and confidence in performing everyday movements.

Remember that functional fitness is about making your body better suited for daily life tasks. As you become more proficient in these exercises, you'll be better prepared to handle various physical challenges with ease and reduced risk of injury.

9

Recovery and Injury Prevention

Techniques for proper recovery, including rest days and injury prevention strategies:

1. Muscle Repair and Growth:

During intense exercise, especially strength training, your muscles undergo micro-tears. Recovery time allows your body to repair these micro-tears, making your muscles stronger and more resilient. This process is essential for muscle growth and increased strength.

2. Inflammation Reduction:

Exercise can lead to inflammation in your muscles and joints. Adequate recovery time helps reduce this inflammation and prevents chronic issues like overuse injuries.

3. Energy Restoration:

Intense workouts deplete your body's energy stores, including glycogen (stored glucose). Recovery time allows your body to replenish these energy reserves, ensuring you have the required fuel for your next workout.

4. Hormonal Balance:

Exercise can temporarily disrupt hormonal balance, especially stress hormones like cortisol. Sufficient recovery time helps restore hormonal equilibrium, which is crucial for overall health.

5. Central Nervous System (CNS) Recovery:

Intense workouts stress your CNS. Recovery time allows your nervous system to recuperate, ensuring optimal coordination and muscle function during subsequent workouts.

6. Prevention of Overtraining:

Failing to provide adequate recovery time can lead to overtraining syndrome. This can result in fatigue, decreased performance, increased injury risk, and even mental burnout.

Recovery Strategies:

- **Rest Days:** Schedule regular rest days where you engage in lighter activities or complete rest. Your body needs time to repair and rejuvenate.

- **Active Recovery**: Engage in light activities like walking, swimming, or yoga on rest days. This promotes blood flow and helps with muscle relaxation.

- **Hydration and Nutrition**: Proper hydration and a balanced diet rich in protein and nutrients aid in muscle repair and replenishing energy stores.

- **Sleep**: Quality sleep is essential for recovery. It's during sleep that growth hormone is released, facilitating muscle repair and overall recovery.

- **Foam Rolling and Stretching:** These practices can help release muscle tension, improve circulation, and increase flexibility.

- **Massage and Bodywork:** Professional massage or self-massage techniques can promote relaxation, reduce muscle soreness, and enhance recovery.

- **Cold and Heat Therapy:** Alternating between cold (ice baths) and heat (saunas) can improve circulation and reduce inflammation.

- **Stress Management**: Psychological stress can impact physical recovery. Engage in stress-relief techniques like meditation or deep breathing.

Individualization:

Recovery needs can vary from person to person based on factors like fitness level, age, intensity of exercise, and overall health. Listening to your body and adjusting your recovery strategies accordingly is essential.

Injury Prevention:

1. **Warm-Up and Cool-Down:**

- **Warm-Up:** A proper warm-up gradually increases your heart rate and blood flow to your muscles. This prepares your body for more intense activity and reduces the risk of muscle strains and joint injuries. A warm-up might include light cardiovascular exercises like jogging, jumping jacks, or cycling, followed by dynamic stretches that mimic the movements you'll be doing during your workout.

- **Cool-Down**: Cooling down after a workout helps your body transition from high-intensity activity to a resting state. It gradually lowers your heart rate and reduces the risk of dizziness or fainting. A cool-down typically involves gentle stretching and slower-paced movements.

2. **Proper Technique**:
   - Using correct form during exercises is crucial. Poor technique can lead to strains, sprains, and other injuries. Before adding weights or intensity, ensure you have mastered the proper form of each exercise. If you're unsure, consider seeking guidance from a fitness professional.

3. **Progressive Overload:**
   - Gradually increasing the weight, resistance, or intensity of your workouts is important for building strength and fitness. However, making sudden or excessive jumps can lead to injuries. Progress gradually to give your muscles, joints, and connective tissues time to adapt.

4. **Cross-Training:**
   - Engaging in a variety of exercises can prevent overuse injuries. For example, if you're primarily a runner, consider adding strength

training, swimming, or yoga to your routine. This gives specific muscle groups a chance to recover while still staying active.

5. **Listen to Your Body:**

- Pain is your body's way of signalling that something is wrong. Ignoring pain and pushing through it can lead to serious injuries. Learn to differentiate between normal muscle fatigue and pain that indicates potential harm.

6. **Flexibility and Mobility:**

- Good flexibility and joint mobility reduce the risk of strains and sprains. Incorporate dynamic stretches into your warm-up and static stretches into your cool-down. Regular flexibility work can also improve your overall athletic performance.

7. **Rest and Recovery:**

- Adequate rest is vital for recovery and injury prevention. Muscles need time to repair and grow stronger after intense workouts. Make sure to schedule regular rest days into your training routine.

8. **Balanced Training:**

- Ensure that your training program is well-rounded. Strengthen opposing muscle groups to maintain balance around joints. For example, if you work on your quadriceps, also work on your hamstrings to prevent imbalances that could lead to injury.

9. **Proper Footwear and Equipment**:

- Wearing appropriate footwear that provides proper support and fits well can prevent injuries, especially for activities like running or weightlifting. Additionally, using well-maintained equipment reduces the risk of accidents.

10. **Hydration and Nutrition:**

- Staying hydrated and consuming a balanced diet supports muscle function and recovery, reducing the risk of fatigue-related injuries.

10

Long-Term Progression and Maintenance

1: **Progressive Overload:**

Let's say you start your strength training journey by performing squats with a barbell using 50 pounds. After a few weeks, you find that doing 3 sets of 10 repetitions has become relatively easy. To apply progressive overload:

- **Increase the Weight**: You could increase the weight to 55 pounds for your squats. This added resistance challenges your muscles and stimulates further growth.

- **Increase Repetitions**: Instead of 10 reps, you could aim for 12 reps with the same weight. This added volume also contributes to muscle adaptation.

2: **Periodization:**

Imagine you've been consistently working out for a year, and you want to prevent plateauing. You decide to implement a periodization approach:

- **Hypertrophy Phase (4 weeks):** During this phase, your goal is muscle growth. You focus on moderate weights and higher repetitions. For instance, you could do 3 sets of 8-12 reps for each exercise.

- **Strength Phase (4 weeks):** In this phase, you prioritize lifting heavier weights with lower reps. You might do 4 sets of 5-6 reps for compound exercises like bench press and deadlift.

- **Power Phase (4 weeks):** This phase emphasizes explosive movements and speed. You incorporate exercises like box jumps and medicine ball throws.

3: <u>Varying Exercises</u>:

As you progress, it's essential to introduce exercise variations to target muscles from different angles. For instance:

- Instead of traditional push-ups, you can do incline push-ups to challenge your upper chest.

- Swap regular lunges for lateral lunges to engage your inner and outer thighs.

- Transition from standard planks to side planks to work on your obliques and core stability.

4: **Adapting to Age and Lifestyle Changes:**

Let's say you're in your 50s, and you've been following a specific routine for a while. However, you're experiencing some joint stiffness. To adopt:

- You might incorporate more dynamic warm-up exercises and focus on joint mobility drills before your workouts.

- Consider reducing the frequency of high-impact exercises and incorporating more low-impact options like swimming or cycling to protect your joints.

5: **<u>Injury Prevention and Management:</u>**

Imagine you start feeling discomfort in your shoulder during overhead presses. Instead of pushing through:

- Lower the weight or switch to a different shoulder exercise that doesn't cause pain.

- Incorporate exercises to strengthen the muscles supporting your shoulder joint, such as rows and rotator cuff exercises.

6: **<u>Enjoyment and Variation</u>**

If you're finding your routine monotonous, it's time to inject some variety:

- Instead of traditional weightlifting, you could try a circuit-style workout that includes bodyweight exercises, kettlebell swings, and resistance band work.

- Consider exploring recreational activities like hiking, rock climbing, or dancing to keep things exciting and active.

Remember, long-term progress and maintenance in strength training require a combination of strategy, consistency, adaptation, and a commitment to lifelong fitness. The key is to listen to your body, stay engaged, and continue challenging yourself within safe and healthy parameters.

Guidelines for progressing your strength training routine over time and maintaining results:

1. **Start Where You Are:** When beginning a strength training routine, it's important to start at a level that matches your current fitness and strength level. This not only prevents injury but also provides a solid foundation for future progress.

2. **Gradually Increase Intensity**: As your body adapts to your initial routine, you need to gradually increase the intensity of your workouts. This can be done by adding more weight, increasing the number of repetitions, or adjusting other variables. The principle of progressive overload is at play here, and it's the key to continued improvement.

3. **Set Clear Goals**: Define specific, measurable goals for your strength training. Whether it's lifting a certain amount of weight, achieving a certain number of repetitions, or mastering a particular exercise, having clear goals gives you direction and motivation.

4. **Use Different Training Techniques**: Incorporate a variety of training techniques to keep your workouts challenging and engaging. This can include techniques like supersets, drop sets, pyramids, and circuit training. These methods can help you break through plateaus and stimulate muscle growth.

5. **Implement Periodization**: Periodization involves dividing your training into distinct phases, each with a specific focus and intensity level. For instance, you might have a strength-building phase followed by a higher-repetition phase for muscle endurance. This strategy prevents plateaus and reduces the risk of overtraining.

6. **Keep Records**: Maintain a detailed record of your workouts, including the exercises, sets, reps, and weights used. This allows you to track your progress over time and make informed decisions about when and how to increase the intensity.

7. **Increase Weight Safely:** When adding more weight to your exercises, prioritize proper form and technique. Gradually increase the weight in small increments to avoid straining your muscles and joints.

8. **Monitor Recovery:** Adequate recovery is essential for progress. Make sure you're getting enough sleep, managing stress, and allowing your muscles time to heal between intense workouts.

9. **Incorporate Deload Weeks**: Periodically, incorporate deload weeks where you reduce the intensity and volume of your workouts. This gives your body a chance to recover and reduces the risk of burnout.

10. **Nutrition Matters:** Proper nutrition supports your strength training efforts. Consume enough protein to aid in muscle repair and growth, and ensure you're getting a balanced diet to fuel your workouts.

11. **Stay Flexible:** Be willing to adapt your routine based on how your body responds. If you experience fatigue, persistent soreness, or other signs of overtraining, it's important to adjust your plan.

12. **Celebrate Achievements**: Acknowledge and celebrate your progress along the way. Whether it's hitting a weightlifting milestone or completing a challenging exercise, recognizing your achievements can boost your motivation.

13. **Long-Term Mindset**: Understand that strength training is a long-term commitment. Results may not be immediate, but with consistent effort, you will see improvements over time.

Remember, the journey of progressing and maintaining results in strength training is a continuous process. It requires dedication, patience, and a willingness to adapt your approach as your body changes and responds to the training. Consulting with fitness professionals can also provide valuable guidance tailored to your individual needs.

11

Conclusion

As you reach the final pages of "Ageless Strength," it's time to reflect on the transformative journey you've undertaken. This book was never just about exercises; it's about discovering the immense reservoirs of strength that lie within you, regardless of your age. You've embarked on a path that defies the constraints of time, proving that strength is not bound by the calendar but nurtured by dedication, resilience, and belief in your potential.

Throughout this book, you've learned that age is not an impediment; it's a backdrop to a story of constant evolution. You've harnessed the power of foundational exercises, building a solid base that allowed you to transcend limitations. From daily routines to the harmonious integration of cardiovascular fitness and strength training, you've reshaped not just your physique but your perspective on what's achievable.

Yet, "Ageless Strength" isn't just about the physical aspects. It's about reclaiming your vitality, reigniting the flame of youthfulness that burns deep within. You've honed your core, not just the muscles but the core of your identity – a person who embraces challenges, who persists when the going gets tough, and who values health as an essential currency of life.

As you've delved into the pages on recovery and injury prevention, you've realized that self-care isn't selfish; it's a prerequisite for sustained progress. Just as a muscle grows stronger during rest, your understanding of the value of balance has grown stronger, and you've embraced the wisdom of honouring both effort and rejuvenation.

And now, as you stand at the intersection of completion and continuation, remember that this journey doesn't culminate here. Your ageless strength is an ongoing symphony, with each day offering a new note to add to the harmony. The conclusion of this book marks the commencement of a life enriched by strength, vitality, and the unwavering knowledge that your potential is boundless.

Let this conclusion be a commencement—a stepping stone towards the life you've envisioned, one where age is no longer a factor that defines your limits, but a testament to the resilience of your spirit. As you close this book, remember that your story is far from over. It's a story of perseverance, transformation, and unceasing growth—an ageless tale of strength.

Embrace it. Live it. Celebrate your ageless strength.

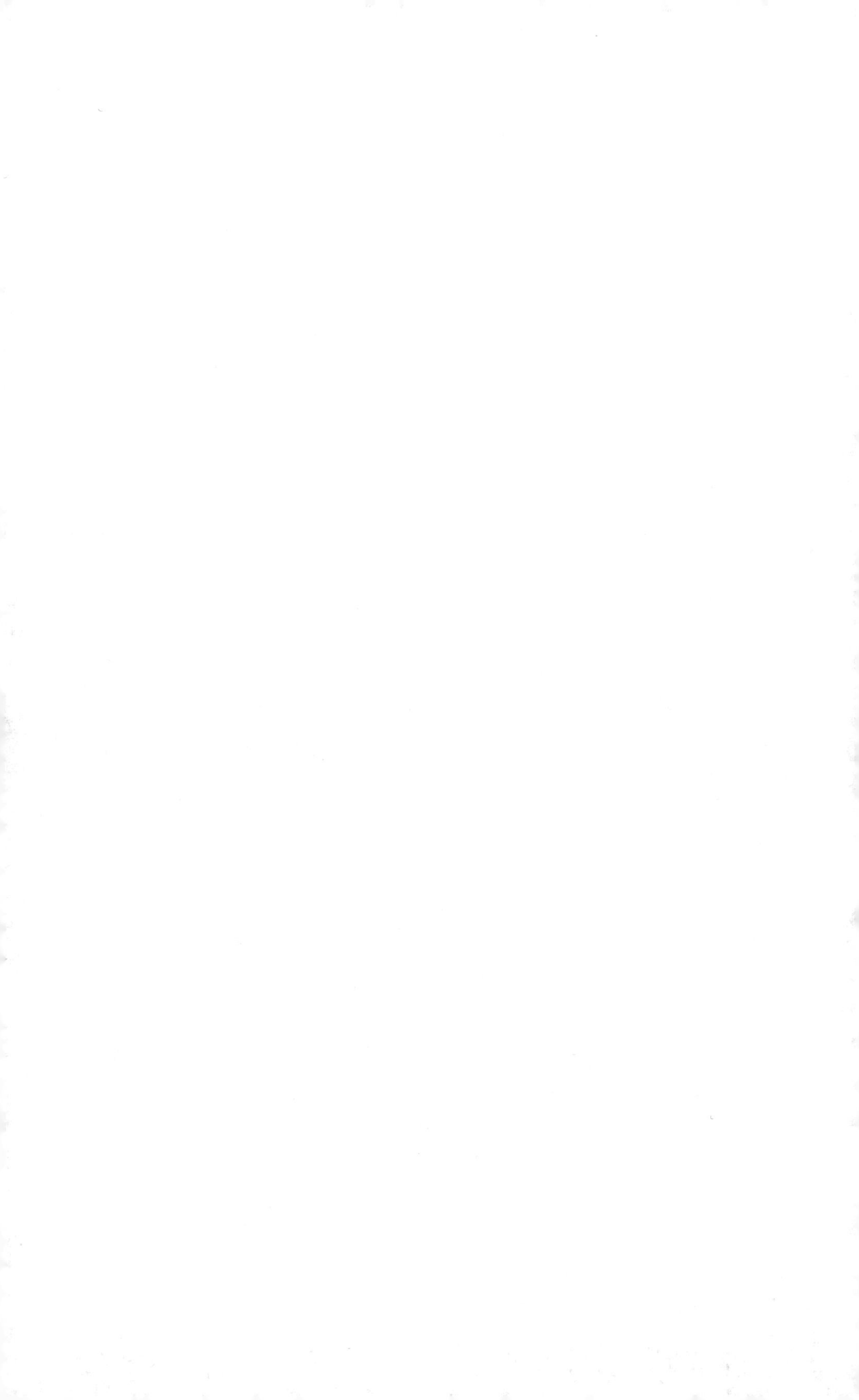